UNDERSTANDING

GLUCOSAMINE

AND BENEFITS

Your Ultimate Handbook To Grasping The Major Targets, Focus, And Key Point For Joint Health And Overall Well-Being

DR. LACEY MICHELLE

Disclaimer:

The information provided in this book is for general informational purposes only and is not intended as medical advice.

Readers are encouraged to consult with a qualified healthcare professional for any health concerns or questions.

Contents

About The Book

Introducing you to the world of glucosamine, a well-liked dietary supplement with potential benefits for improved joint health and mobility. We explore all aspects of glucosamine in this extensive book, including its history, health advantages, scientific basis, and future possibilities. Come along with us as we uncover the mysteries of this amazing supplement on a journey of discovery and comprehension.

Getting to Know Glucosamine

We build the groundwork in the first chapter by responding to the most important queries about glutathione. What is glucosamine, how is it made, and what are some possible advantages? We also look at the many kinds of glucosamine supplements that are sold.

Glucosamine and Joint Health

Here, we highlight the critical function that glucosamine fulfills in maintaining joint health. We go over common joint ailments including osteoarthritis and arthritis and how glucosamine can be a useful tool in treating these problems.

The Functions of Glucosamine

We explore the complex mechanisms of glucosamine in this chapter. Find out how glucosamine supports joint lubrication and general joint function by interacting with cartilage and synovial fluid.

Selecting the Appropriate Glucosamine Supplement

Selecting the ideal glucosamine supplement might be difficult. To help you make an informed choice, we offer information on the various available forms, important considerations, and possible adverse effects.

Evidence and Research from Science

This chapter delves into the scientific basis of glucosamine. We examine safety, efficacy, and clinical research in addition to exploring the arguments and controversies surrounding this supplement.

Glucosamine in Combination with Other Supplements

Learn how glucosamine frequently works in conjunction with other supplements to improve joint support and general health, such as chondroitin, collagen, MSM (Methylsulfonylmethane), and omega-3 fatty acids.

Glucosamine for Particular Populations, This chapter provides an overview of

Glucosamine's adaptability and diversity by examining how it serves a variety of demographic groups, including pets, sports, and the elderly.

Advice on Taking Supplemental Glucosamine

Get insightful advice on how to utilize glucosamine efficiently. We address issues like appropriate dosage, possible interactions, safety measures, and alerts to guarantee a positive and risk-free experience.

Anecdotes and Firsthand Accounts

Hear about the success stories and personal accounts of people who have used glucosamine in their lives. Their experiences and conclusions provide insightful information and motivation.

Glucosamine's Future

Discover what lies ahead for glucosamine as we examine recent findings, developing patterns, and possible inventions. Learn about the fascinating opportunities that await in the field of joint health.

In summary

By the time this book comes to an end, we will have synthesized all of the information and understanding we have gained from studying glutathione.

We trust that you now possess a more profound comprehension of this extraordinary supplement, its capabilities, and its role in the realm of health and well-being.

This book seeks to provide you with a comprehensive understanding of glucosamine, an important dietary supplement, whether you're looking for joint relief or are just interested in the science behind it.

CHAPTER ONE

Glucosamine: What Is It?

Glucosamine is a naturally occurring substance that is mostly found in cartilage, the connective tissue that surrounds and cushions joints in the human body.

It is essential for the development and upkeep of strong joint cartilage. As a sugar with an amino group, glucosamine is categorized as an amino sugar.

It is a constituent of several structural components in the body.

It is frequently taken as a dietary supplement to maintain joint health, especially in diseases where cartilage degradation is a major issue, such as osteoarthritis.

Glucosamine Synopsis

There are several different types of glucosamine supplements on the market, such as glucosamine hydrochloride, glucosamine sulfate, and N-acetyl-glucosamine. People who want to reduce joint discomfort, increase joint mobility, and possibly even slow down the advancement of joint-related illnesses frequently utilize these supplements. Glucosamine supplements are typically taken orally and may be found in many pharmacies and health food stores without a prescription.

Natural Glucosamine Sources

Although food sources can naturally offer glucosamine, the amount consumed through diet alone might not be enough to produce the therapeutic results seen with supplementation.

Crab, lobster, and shrimp are examples of shellfish that are very high in glucosamine. Furthermore, because cartilage breaks down during boiling, bone broth—which is created by simmering animal bones and connective tissues—may include trace levels of glucosamine.

While some people may include these foods in their diet to help with joint health, taking glucosamine pills is frequently a more dependable and straightforward way to get the nutrients.

The Molecular Basis Of Glucosamine

The idea that glucosamine supplements can give the body more building blocks to help cartilage health and repair is the main reason for their use.

The following are some salient features of glucosamine science:

Cartilage Health: Cartilage serves as a shock absorber and contributes to the smooth motion of joints, making it essential to joint function.

Osteoarthritis is one ailment where cartilage gradually deteriorates, causing pain and decreased mobility.

Glucosamine is frequently used in the treatment of osteoarthritis because it is thought to aid in the maintenance and repair of cartilage.

Glucosamine is hypothesized to provide chondro protective properties, which could shield cartilage from further deterioration.

It has been suggested that glucosamine aids in the stimulation of the synthesis of proteoglycans and glycosaminoglycans, two vital constituents of robust cartilage.

Anti-Inflammatory Properties: According to certain research, glucosamine may have minor anti-inflammatory properties that may relieve joint discomfort brought on by diseases like osteoarthritis.

Glucosamine pills may help ease discomfort by lowering inflammation.

Clinical Evidence: There is still discussion and study about the efficacy of glucosamine supplementation.

In instances of mild to severe osteoarthritis, in particular, several clinical trials have demonstrated beneficial outcomes in terms of lowering joint pain and enhancing joint function.

Nevertheless, there have been conflicting findings, and not all research has shown meaningful advantages. Individual differences exist in how each person reacts to glucosamine.

Glucosamine is a naturally occurring substance that may be obtained from specific food sources and the body.

 It is mostly taken as a dietary supplement to help maintain healthy joints and treat diseases like osteoarthritis.

The ability of glucosamine to preserve and protect cartilage, lessen inflammation, and ease joint discomfort is the basis of its scientific basis.

Even though there have been some studies that show it to be effective, there is inconsistent data, and each person's experience may differ.

Before beginning any supplement regimen, it is best to speak with a healthcare provider, particularly if you have underlying joint problems or are thinking about using glucosamine for therapeutic purposes.

CHAPTER TWO

Glucosamine Supplement Types

There are numerous varieties of glucosamine supplements on the market, each with special qualities and possible advantages.

The main purposes of these supplements are to promote joint health and reduce osteoarthritis symptoms, which are caused by a prevalent degenerative joint disease. Knowing the distinctions between these kinds will assist people in making well-informed decisions regarding which one could be best for their particular needs.

Sulfate Of Glucosamine

One of the most popular kinds of glucosamine supplements is glucosamine sulfate.

It is made up of glucosamine molecules bonded to sulfate, an element the body naturally contains.

Because it may aid in the creation of cartilage and joint fluid, this sulfate form is regarded to be useful in relieving the symptoms of osteoarthritis.

Numerous clinical studies have examined the advantages of glucosamine sulfate, and some have shown that it can help people with osteoarthritis feel less pain and move more easily in their joints.

For people looking for combined support, this kind is frequently advised.

Hydrochloride Glucosamine (HCL)

Another type of glucosamine supplement is called glucosamine hydrochloride, or glucosamine HCL. It is devoid of sulfate molecules, in contrast to glucosamine sulfate. Glucosamine coupled to hydrochloride is what makes up glucosamine HCL, on the other hand.

Some people prefer glucosamine HCL because of its higher glucosamine content by weight, even though it doesn't contain sulfate.

For people who react poorly to glucosamine sulfate or who are sensitive to sulfur, this version might be more appropriate. On the other hand, glucosamine HCL has not been the subject of as much investigation as glucosamine sulfate.

Acetyl-Glucosamine N-Acetyl

Another form of glucosamine supplementation is called N-Acetyl Glucosamine, or NAG for short.

It is glucosamine in a modified form with an acetyl group added. This alteration may have an impact on how the body absorbs and uses NAG.

While glucosamine sulfate or glucosamine HCL are more frequently used for joint health, NAG is occasionally added to supplements due to its possible involvement in promoting the health of connective tissues, such as cartilage and mucous membranes. The acetyl group may improve NAG's bioavailability and absorption.

Blending Formulas

Certain glucosamine supplements are made up of blends of various forms of glucosamine, frequently consisting of glucosamine sulfate, glucosamine HCL, and NAG.

The purpose of these combination formulas is to provide a wider range of possible advantages. By addressing several facets of joint health, they offer a more all-encompassing method of treating osteoarthritis symptoms.

Those who wish to investigate the possible synergistic effects of several glucosamine types can use combination formulations.

N-acetyl glucosamine (NAG), glucosamine sulfate, glucosamine HCL, and combination formulations are among the different kinds of glucosamine supplements available.

Which kind to utilize will depend on the person seeking joint support's particular needs, preferences, and sensitivities.

Before beginning any supplement regimen, it is imperative to speak with a healthcare provider. They can offer advice on the best form and dose based on a person's unique situation and health objectives.

CHAPTER THREE

Osteoarthritis and Joint Health: Glucosamine is a naturally occurring substance that is important for maintaining joint health, especially when osteoarthritis is present.

Osteoarthritis is a common degenerative joint disease that causes pain, stiffness, and limited joint motion due to the slow destruction of cartilage.

As a vital component of cartilage, glucosamine is thought to support joint health by assisting in the upkeep and repair of this connective tissue.

It is frequently taken as a supplement to assist in reducing osteoarthritis symptoms.

Glucosamine's effectiveness in treating osteoarthritis has been the subject of numerous investigations and clinical trials. There is a body of research indicating that glucosamine supplementation may offer relief from joint pain and stiffness, despite the relatively inconsistent results.

It is believed that glucosamine's capacity to promote cartilage synthesis and shield pre-existing cartilage from more harm is the mechanism underlying this advantage.

This may help those with osteoarthritis have less discomfort and better joint function.

Cartilage Repair And Maintenance:

Glucosamine's main job is to keep the smooth, rubbery tissue that covers the ends of bones in a joint structurally intact.

As a cushion, cartilage facilitates easy joint motion and absorbs shock during activity. Cartilage injury can occur as a result of aging, wear and tear, and joint traumas over time.

It is thought that cartilage regeneration and maintenance are critically dependent on glucosamine.

Apart from its ability to decelerate the deterioration of cartilage, glucosamine also possesses the capacity to incite the creation of proteoglycans and collagen, two crucial constituents of cartilage.

Glucosamine helps build and repair damaged cartilage by encouraging the synthesis of these structural molecules, which further supports joint health.

Supporting the maintenance of cartilage is especially important for people who want to heal from joint injuries or maintain healthy joints.

Reduction of Inflammation In diseases like osteoarthritis, inflammation plays a major role in joint discomfort and destruction.

Some research suggests that glucosamine has anti-inflammatory qualities, which may help lessen joint inflammatory processes.

The release of enzymes that degrade cartilage and produce discomfort and edema can result from inflammation.

Because of its ability to lower inflammation, glucosamine may potentially provide further relief for those who suffer from joint problems.

Despite not having the same anti-inflammatory effect as non-steroidal anti-inflammatory medicines (NSAIDs), glucosamine is nevertheless regarded as a more natural and safe option for long-term use.

Glucosamine offers an integrated approach to joint health management by treating the structural and inflammatory elements of joint health.

Possibility for Additional Health Benefits Glucosamine may offer additional health benefits beyond its main function in joint health, according to new research.

It may help reduce inflammation and maintain blood vessel health, which is why some research has looked into its possible impacts on cardiovascular health.

Furthermore, glucosamine's potential to enhance gut health and lower the risk of inflammatory bowel illnesses has been studied.

It's important to remember, though, that additional study is required to determine the scope of these possible advantages and their mechanisms.

Other than joint-related problems, glucosamine shouldn't be taken as a stand-alone medication without first speaking with a medical practitioner.

It is often known that glucosamine supplements can improve joint health, especially when osteoarthritis is present.

They are a well-liked option for people looking for a natural and comprehensive approach to joint care because of their capacity to assist cartilage repair and maintenance, lower inflammation, and maybe provide other health advantages.

However, before beginning any supplementation regimen, it is imperative to speak with a healthcare physician because different people may respond differently to glucosamine and it may not be a good fit for everyone.

CHAPTER FOUR

Dosage And Usage Of Glucosamine

A naturally occurring substance present in good cartilage, glucosamine is critical for preserving the flexibility and health of joints.

It is a well-liked dietary supplement that many people take to relieve osteoarthritis and joint pain. There are a few important considerations to make when thinking about the dosage and use of glucosamine.

Suggested Dosages:

Depending on the particular kind of glucosamine being taken, different dosages may be advised. Glucosamine hydrochloride and glucosamine sulfate are the most widely used types. Doses typically consist of two or three doses, ranging from 1,500 to 2,000 milligrams per day. That being said, each person's ideal dosage may vary, so it's best to speak with a healthcare provider before beginning any supplement routine.

Some people may need to take glucosamine supplements for a longer amount of time to see the full advantages, and it may take several weeks for their effectiveness to become apparent.

Furthermore, it's critical to adhere to the directions on the product label because glucosamine concentrations might vary throughout manufacturers and formulas.

Safety Measures:

When taken at authorized quantities, most persons are thought to be safe when using glucosamine.

Like any vitamin, though, some people may experience negative effects from it. Mild gastrointestinal side effects like upset stomach, diarrhea, or nausea are common. The supplement's temporary adverse effects can be reduced by taking it with food.

One crucial thing to keep in mind is that glucosamine is frequently made from the shells of shellfish, which means that people who are allergic to shellfish should not take it.

In certain situations, glucosamine from a source other than shellfish can be required.

Furthermore, you should speak with your doctor before beginning a glucosamine program if you are pregnant, nursing, have diabetes or are on blood thinners.

These people may need to watch their dosage or exercise caution because of possible interactions and effects on blood sugar levels.

Different populations may respond differently to glucosamine supplements.

For instance, glucosamine has been demonstrated to lessen pain and enhance joint function in patients with mild to moderate osteoarthritis, which may make them more likely to benefit from it.

In cases of severe osteoarthritis, the advantages might not be as noticeable.

Furthermore, it's important to remember that glucosamine may work better in conjunction with chondroitin sulfate, another nutritional supplement that's frequently taken for joint health.

Clinical trials have demonstrated the potential of this combination to reduce osteoarthritis symptoms.

Supplementing with glucosamine may be beneficial for elderly people, as they are more likely to experience joint problems.

To find the best dosage and make sure glucosamine won't interfere with any other medications they may be taking, seniors should talk about using glucosamine with their healthcare professional.

As a supplement, glucosamine has the potential to improve joint health and reduce osteoarthritis symptoms.

 To ensure safe and effective use, it is always advisable to consult with a healthcare provider, taking into account any unique needs or potential contraindications based on an individual's health profile.

However, determining the appropriate dosage and usage requires consideration of individual factors.

CHAPTER FIVE

Supplemental Glucosamine Versus Prescription Medication

Prescription drugs and glucosamine supplements are two alternatives for treating joint-related disorders, especially osteoarthritis. Although they both aim to reduce joint discomfort and increase mobility, they are very different from one another in several important ways.

A Comparative Study

Glucosamine sulfate, a naturally occurring substance present in some foods and our bodies, is the ingredient in glucosamine supplements.

It is typically manufactured synthetically or obtained from shellfish.

On the other hand, pharmaceutical pharmaceuticals that are particularly made to target inflammation and pain are prescription medications for joint pain, such as corticosteroids or nonsteroidal anti-inflammatory drugs (NSAIDs).

Their respective modes of action are among the main differences between the two. It is thought that glucosamine functions by encouraging the manufacture of cartilage-forming molecules, which may inhibit the deterioration of joint tissues.

Conversely, prescription drugs do not directly address cartilage regeneration; instead, their primary goals are pain management and inflammation reduction.

A crucial distinction is safety. Supplementing with glucosamine is typically regarded as safe, with the majority of adverse effects being minor stomach problems.

On the other hand, a variety of adverse consequences are possible with prescription drugs, such as heart difficulties, gastrointestinal disorders, and the risk of addiction or dependency, particularly with long-term opioid usage.

Cost should also be taken into account. Since glucosamine pills are sold over the counter, many people find them to be a more cost-effective option.

Prescription drugs, on the other hand, can be significantly more costly, particularly if insurance does not cover them.

Which Is Better: Glucosamine or

The choice between prescription drugs and glucosamine supplements is influenced by several variables, such as the particular ailment being treated, the patient's general health, and personal preferences. When taking glucosamine might be a better option:

Early-stage Osteoarthritis: Glucosamine may be a good place to start if you have mild to moderate osteoarthritis and would like to treat your symptoms conservatively.

Preventative Measures: If an individual is more susceptible to joint issues owing to age, genetics, or past accidents, they may want to consider taking glucosamine supplements as a preventive approach to promote joint health.

Minimal Side Effects: Glucosamine is usually well-tolerated, so if you're worried about possible side effects or would rather take a more natural approach, this is a good option.

Affordability: Glucosamine supplements are a sensible choice for people on a tight budget because they are frequently more affordable.

It's important to remember that glucosamine's effectiveness varies from person to person and that results can not show up for weeks or even months. As a result, it could not offer severe joint pain relief right away.

Possible Relationships

It is crucial to be aware of any possible interactions with other medications or medical conditions when thinking about taking glucosamine supplements. Given that it has a slight blood-thinning effect of its own, glucosamine may interact with blood-thinning drugs.

If you use any of these drugs or have bleeding issues, you should speak with a doctor before beginning glucosamine.

To prevent allergic reactions, people who are allergic to shellfish should choose a vegetarian or synthetic glucosamine source.

If taking glucosamine, diabetics should regularly check their blood sugar levels as glucosamine may interact with diabetes drugs and influence blood sugar levels.

The choice between prescription pharmaceuticals and glucosamine supplements is influenced by several factors, such as the type of joint problem, personal preferences, and possible drug interactions. Always seek the advice of a medical expert to ascertain the best course of action for your particular circumstances.

Selecting the Correct Glucosamine Supplement might be a Crucial Choice for People Hoping to Relieve Joint Pain and Enhance Joint Health.

A naturally occurring substance in good cartilage, glucosamine is essential for preserving joint function. It is frequently taken as a dietary supplement to promote joint health and lessen osteoarthritis symptoms.

But not every glucosamine supplement is made equally. There are many things to take into account to make an informed decision, such as reading labels, determining purity, and rating quality.

Factors To Consider:

There are several things to think about when thinking about taking a glucosamine supplement. Consult a qualified physician or other healthcare practitioner first. They can offer insightful information about your unique requirements and assist in determining whether a glucosamine supplement is suitable for your health.

In addition, they can provide advice on the appropriate form and dosage of glucosamine, including N-acetyl glucosamine, glucosamine hydrochloride, and glucosamine sulfate.

When choosing a glucosamine supplement, other factors to consider are age, current health issues, and any potential allergies or sensitivities.

For different people, different formulations and delivery systems—such as tablets, capsules, or liquid forms—might be more appropriate. For maximum benefit, it could occasionally be required to take glucosamine along with other supplements for joint health, such as chondroitin or MSM.

Reading Labels:

It's important to know what you're putting into your body when it comes to glucosamine supplements.

The type of glucosamine used, the amount per serving, and any other components should all be clearly stated on the label.

The kind of glucosamine is important since different types have different qualities and might work better for particular uses.

For example, glucosamine hydrochloride is mostly utilized to improve joint health, but glucosamine sulfate is frequently used for osteoarthritis.

Another important factor to consider is the dosage per serving. Verify if the glucosamine dosage in the supplement is suitable and efficient. It's also critical to look for any allergens, fillers, or additives that might not be good for your health or fit within your dietary limitations.

A trustworthy producer must guarantee label transparency and include a list of all ingredients.

Quality and Purity: A glucosamine supplement's efficacy and safety can be significantly impacted by its quality and purity.

Selecting goods from reputable companies with a solid track record of creating high-quality supplements is advised.

Seek supplements that have been subjected to independent testing, as this guarantees an additional degree of transparency and quality control.

When it comes to the supplement's lack of pollutants or other impurities, purity is equally important.

The product must be free of toxins, heavy metals, and other dangerous materials to guarantee that your health won't be jeopardized.

As some supplements contain glucosamine derived from shellfish, allergen testing should be part of the purity considerations for people who have a shellfish allergy.

It is important to carefully consider several factors when choosing a glucosamine supplement, including your specific health needs, the type of glucosamine you take, the information on the label, and the product's quality and purity. Consulting a healthcare professional and conducting thorough research can help individuals make an informed decision that best suits their joint health goals and overall well-being.

By paying attention to these factors, you can maximize the potential benefits of glucosamine supplementation while minimizing potential risks and side effects.

CHAPTER SIX

Combining Glucosamine With Other Supplements

Combining glucosamine with other supplements is a common practice aimed at enhancing the potential benefits of this popular dietary supplement for joint health. Glucosamine is a natural compound found in the body and is commonly used as a dietary supplement to support joint health and alleviate symptoms of osteoarthritis.

However, it is often used in conjunction with other supplements to maximize its effectiveness. Here, we explore the concepts of combining glucosamine with various other supplements, including chondroitin, MSM (Methylsulfonylmethane), omega-3 fatty acids, vitamin D, and calcium.

Chondroitin

Chondroitin is often paired with glucosamine in joint health supplements. It is a natural compound found in cartilage and is thought to work synergistically with glucosamine. Chondroitin helps to maintain the structural integrity of cartilage and inhibits the enzymes that break it down.

When combined with glucosamine, these two compounds may provide a more comprehensive approach to joint health. Studies suggest that this combination can offer greater pain relief and improved joint function than either supplement alone. However, the effectiveness of glucosamine and chondroitin in combination can vary from person to person.

MSM (Methylsulfonylmethane)

MSM, or Methylsulfonylmethane, is a naturally occurring sulfur compound found in certain foods and used as a dietary supplement for various purposes, including joint health.

It is often combined with glucosamine because sulfur is a key component in the production of collagen, a crucial protein in the structure of joints and connective tissues. When used alongside glucosamine, MSM is believed to promote joint flexibility and reduce inflammation.

Some studies suggest that this combination can alleviate osteoarthritis symptoms. However, more research is needed to establish its efficacy conclusively.

Omega-3 fatty acids, primarily found in fish oil supplements, are known for their anti-inflammatory properties and potential benefits for joint health.

When combined with glucosamine, omega-3 fatty acids can provide a multifaceted approach to reducing joint pain and inflammation.

Omega-3s help by reducing the production of inflammatory molecules and can enhance the overall effectiveness of glucosamine.

This combination may be particularly beneficial for individuals with inflammatory joint conditions, such as rheumatoid arthritis. However, the optimal dosages and specific benefits of this combination can vary among individuals.

Vitamin D and calcium are essential nutrients for maintaining healthy bones and joints.

Vitamin D helps the body absorb calcium, which is necessary for bone and joint health. Combining these two nutrients with glucosamine can provide a holistic approach to support not only joint health but also bone health.

Ensuring adequate levels of vitamin D and calcium is essential, especially for individuals at risk of osteoporosis and osteoarthritis. However, it's important to be mindful of the recommended daily intake of these nutrients, as excessive supplementation can lead to adverse effects.

combining glucosamine with other supplements is a strategy aimed at enhancing its potential benefits for joint health.

These combinations can provide a more comprehensive approach to alleviate joint pain, improve joint function, and reduce inflammation. While research supports the efficacy of some of these combinations, the outcomes may vary from person to person. It's advisable to consult with a healthcare professional before starting any supplement regimen, as they can guide the most appropriate supplements and dosages based on individual needs and conditions.

Glucosamine And Exercise

Glucosamine is a popular dietary supplement known for its potential benefits in supporting joint health.

It is often sought after by individuals engaging in various forms of exercise, including athletes, fitness enthusiasts, and those looking to maintain an active lifestyle. This article delves into the relationship between glucosamine supplementation and exercise, exploring the joint support it may offer to individuals who engage in physical activity.

Joint Support For Athletes

Athletes, both professional and amateur, subject their joints to rigorous and repetitive stress during their training and competition. This constant wear and tear can lead to joint discomfort and, in some cases, more severe issues like osteoarthritis.

Glucosamine, a naturally occurring compound in the body, is a key component of cartilage, which cushions and protects the joints.

When taken as a supplement, glucosamine is believed to contribute to joint health by supporting the maintenance and repair of cartilage.

For athletes, maintaining healthy joints is crucial to their performance and long-term well-being.

While scientific evidence on the efficacy of glucosamine is mixed, some studies suggest that it may help reduce joint pain and stiffness, particularly in individuals with osteoarthritis.

These potential benefits can be attractive to athletes looking to minimize the negative impacts of intense training on their joints and continue performing at their best.

CHAPTER SEVEN

Glucosamine And Physical Activity

Physical activity is not limited to professional athletes; it includes a wide range of exercises, from weightlifting and running to yoga and recreational sports.

Regardless of the level of intensity, these activities can put a strain on joints. Glucosamine supplements are sometimes considered by those engaged in physical activity as a preventive measure to maintain joint health.

The idea behind glucosamine supplementation is that it may help the body repair and maintain cartilage more effectively, thereby reducing the risk of joint-related problems. This potential preventive aspect of glucosamine can make it appealing to individuals who value their physical well-being and aim to enjoy an active lifestyle for years to come.

Precautions For Intensive Exercise

While glucosamine supplements may offer benefits to those engaging in physical activity, it's essential to exercise caution and consider a few precautions, especially for individuals involved in intensive exercise.

First and foremost, it's advisable to consult a healthcare professional before starting any supplement regimen, as individual responses to glucosamine can vary. They can provide personalized advice and assess whether glucosamine is suitable for your specific needs.

Furthermore, glucosamine supplements are not a magical cure for joint problems, and their effects may take time to manifest.

Therefore, they should not be relied upon as the sole solution for joint health.

 A holistic approach to exercise, including proper warm-ups, cool-downs, and adopting joint-friendly techniques, is essential.

Maintaining a balanced diet and staying hydrated are also key factors in supporting overall joint health.

glucosamine is a dietary supplement that has gained attention for its potential benefits in supporting joint health, making it appealing to athletes and individuals engaged in physical activity.

While it may offer some advantages, it should be approached with caution, and consultation with a healthcare professional is advisable. Ultimately, a well-rounded approach to exercise, including good practices and lifestyle choices, is vital in maintaining joint health and optimizing physical performance.

Glucosamine In Veterinary Medicine

Glucosamine, a naturally occurring compound, has gained popularity in the field of veterinary medicine as a potential therapeutic option for managing joint health in pets.

Much like in human medicine, glucosamine is often used in the treatment of osteoarthritis and other joint-related conditions in animals.

Understanding the application of glucosamine in veterinary medicine involves exploring its benefits, considerations, and the appropriate dosage and administration protocols.

Glucosamine, a compound found in healthy cartilage, is used as a dietary supplement for pets to support joint health and alleviate the symptoms associated with joint disorders, especially in aging animals.

As pets age, the natural production of glucosamine within their bodies may decline, leading to a decrease in cartilage repair and joint lubrication.

This decline can result in conditions like osteoarthritis, which are characterized by joint pain, stiffness, and reduced mobility. Glucosamine supplements are designed to address these issues by providing an exogenous source of this crucial compound.

In veterinary medicine, glucosamine supplements are often available in various forms, including tablets, capsules, liquid formulations, and even treats, making it convenient for pet owners to administer the supplement to their furry companions.

These supplements can be an integral part of a comprehensive approach to managing joint health in pets, alongside proper nutrition, exercise, weight management, and other treatments, as prescribed by veterinarians.

Benefits And Considerations

The use of glucosamine in pets can offer several potential benefits. These include:

Pain Relief: Glucosamine is believed to have anti-inflammatory properties, helping to reduce joint pain and inflammation in pets suffering from osteoarthritis or other joint conditions.

Cartilage Support: Glucosamine provides the building blocks necessary for the repair and maintenance of cartilage in joints, potentially slowing down the degenerative process.

Improved Mobility: By promoting joint health and lubrication, glucosamine may help pets regain or maintain their mobility and activity levels, contributing to a better quality of life.

Minimal Side Effects: Glucosamine supplements typically have a low risk of adverse effects, making them a relatively safe option for long-term use in pets.

However, it's important to consider certain factors when using glucosamine for pets. Firstly, the efficacy of glucosamine supplements may vary among individual animals, and not all pets will respond to treatment in the same way.

Secondly, it's crucial to consult with a veterinarian before starting any glucosamine regimen, as they can assess the specific needs of the pet and provide guidance on the best approach.

The Administration And Dosage

Determining the appropriate dosage and administration of glucosamine for pets is essential to ensure its effectiveness and safety.

Veterinarians play a crucial role in this process, as they can provide personalized recommendations based on the pet's age, size, breed, and the severity of their joint condition.

Generally, glucosamine is administered orally, either as a standalone supplement or as part of a joint health formula.

Typical dosages for dogs may range from 500 to 1,500 milligrams per day, depending on the specific product and the dog's size. Cats may require lower doses, typically around 125 to 250 milligrams daily. However, it's essential to follow the veterinarian's guidance regarding the exact dosage and form of glucosamine.

glucosamine has established itself as a valuable tool in veterinary medicine for supporting joint health in pets. While it offers numerous potential benefits, pet owners should approach its use with consideration and under the guidance of a qualified veterinarian.

Proper dosage and administration are key to ensuring that glucosamine supplements contribute positively to the well-being and comfort of our beloved animal companions.

CHAPTER EIGHT

Future Research And Development

The future of research and developments in the field of glucosamine supplements holds promise for gaining a deeper understanding of their potential benefits and applications. As science continues to advance, researchers are expected to delve further into the mechanisms of action, safety, and efficacy of glucosamine supplementation.

This research will help to refine our understanding of the compound's potential in promoting joint health and addressing other health concerns.

Current Research Trends

Current research trends surrounding glucosamine supplements are multi-faceted. One of the prominent areas of study involves exploring the mechanisms through which glucosamine may exert its effects on joint health. Researchers are investigating the anti-inflammatory properties of glucosamine, as well as its role in cartilage formation and repair.

These studies aim to uncover the precise biological pathways involved in glucosamine's impact on joint function.

Additionally, there is a growing interest in exploring the potential applications of glucosamine beyond joint health.

Some research suggests that glucosamine may have a role in mitigating symptoms of osteoarthritis, while other studies investigate its use in conditions such as inflammatory bowel disease, asthma, and even neurological disorders.

The versatility of glucosamine as a potential therapeutic agent is an intriguing avenue for further exploration.

Potential Applications

The potential applications of glucosamine supplements extend beyond joint health. While their use for alleviating symptoms of osteoarthritis and promoting overall joint function is well-documented, ongoing research is shedding light on additional areas where glucosamine may be beneficial.

For instance, glucosamine's anti-inflammatory properties have led to studies examining its potential in managing inflammatory conditions such as rheumatoid arthritis and inflammatory bowel disease.

These applications could provide new treatment options for individuals suffering from these ailments.

Furthermore, the link between glucosamine and cartilage health has opened up avenues for research into its use in post-injury recovery, particularly in athletes and individuals with sports-related injuries. There is also continuing study into the potential neuroprotective properties of glucosamine, suggesting its utility in illnesses like Alzheimer's disease and other neurodegenerative disorders.

Ongoing Studies

Numerous ongoing investigations are contributing to the corpus of knowledge surrounding glucosamine supplements.

These studies span a wide range of issues, including the assessment of the long-term safety and efficacy of glucosamine, the identification of optimal dosages for particular illnesses, and the potential synergistic effects of glucosamine with other chemicals or therapies.

Additionally, research trials are being done to better study its effectiveness in controlling numerous health conditions, from osteoarthritis to asthma.

Researchers are also concentrating on understanding the pharmacokinetics and bioavailability of glucosamine, which can impact its absorption and effectiveness.

As technology progresses, researchers are increasingly leveraging cutting-edge technologies like as genomics and metabolomics to acquire a more comprehensive knowledge of the molecular interactions and pathways involved.

the future of glucosamine supplement research is distinguished by a holistic strategy that spans varied applications, potential therapeutic benefits, and a fuller understanding of its mechanisms of action. Ongoing investigations and advances in this field are anticipated to offer new insights into the different applications of glucosamine and may pave the way for more tailored and effective therapies for a variety of health issues.

Actual Testimonials

Testimonials from real people can give important information about how well glucosamine supplements work to maintain joint health and reduce the symptoms of diseases like osteoarthritis.

These endorsements frequently originate from people who have personally benefited from glucosamine. Although they can't replace thorough scientific study, they can provide insight into the experiences of persons who have included glucosamine in their daily routines.

Many people who take glucosamine supplements report notable reductions in pain and improvements in joint function. These testimonies frequently emphasize the possibility of improved mobility, decreased stiffness, and an overall rise in their standard of living.

Users talk about their experiences picking up physical activities that they had given up on because of joint pain.

It's crucial to remember that not every testimonial is overwhelmingly positive. Some people might not get the expected advantages or can have negative side effects. These testimonies are also crucial since they clarify the range of reactions to glucosamine. They serve as a reminder that the way glucosamine interacts with our bodies varies greatly according to the individual.

Individual Narratives Of Glucosamine Addicts
People who use glucosamine supplements for various reasons have a wide range of personal anecdotes to share about their experiences.

These tales frequently highlight the variety of ailments that glucosamine can help with, such as osteoarthritis, joint trauma, and maintaining general joint health.

Those who have had osteoarthritis for a long time may talk about their experiences with different forms of treatment, like physical therapy and painkillers.

As an adjunct to these treatments, some people decide to use glucosamine supplements in their regular routines. Their accounts might explain how they gradually saw increases in joint function and decreased discomfort, which improved their quality of life.

Others may relate their experiences taking glucosamine prophylactically to keep their joints healthy and stop the development of diseases like osteoarthritis.

In these situations, users may discuss how they have managed to keep an active lifestyle and lower their chance of developing joint-related problems as they get older.

Tales Of Triumph And Difficulties

Success tales frequently highlight the advantages and enhancements that people who have included glucosamine in their lives have experienced. These success stories demonstrate the supplement's potential advantages by showcasing how well it works to manage joint pain and enhance joint health in general.

People may have less discomfort, more mobility, and improved capacity to partake in their favorite activities.

It's important to understand, though, that not everyone who takes glucosamine supplements has such striking results. Obstacles could be the need for additional therapies, negative effects, or a lack of discernible improvement.

People frequently talk about how little or nothing they have benefited from using glucosamine.

Difficulties may also stem from variables including dosage, length of usage, and the particular brand of glucosamine (glucosamine hydrochloride or glucosamine sulfate) that a person has experimented with.

These insights assist prospective users in realizing that, although glucosamine may be beneficial for certain people, it may not be a panacea.

Conclusion

Real-world endorsements and first-hand accounts from glucosamine users provide insight into the possible advantages and drawbacks of glucosamine supplementation for joint health. These stories have the potential to be enlightening and inspirational. Although the supplement has been shown to improve joint function, reduce pain, and improve quality of life, these anecdotal reports also highlight the variation in individual reactions, potential difficulties, and adverse effects.

It is essential to analyze these testimonies critically and impartially. They shouldn't take the place of clinical advice and scientific research, even though they might provide insightful information and inspiration for people thinking about taking glucosamine supplements. A healthcare professional's advice and an evaluation of peer-reviewed studies regarding the effectiveness of glucosamine are still essential when deciding whether to include it in one's routine. Although firsthand accounts can be instructive, they only make up a small portion of the information needed to fully comprehend the potential advantages and restrictions of glucosamine supplements.

the broader benefits of metabolic health and how it extends beyond weight management to impact your overall health positively.

8.   Your Long-Term Companion: Metabolic Confusion isn't a quick fix; it's a lifestyle. Learn how to navigate challenges, sustain your progress, and cultivate a positive mindset that supports your ongoing success.

> **Get ready to embark on a transformative journey that simplifies the complexities of weight loss and empowers you to achieve the desired results. Are you prepared to make metabolic confusion work for you? Let's begin this exciting adventure together.**

◆ ◆ ◆

CHAPTER 1:

Understanding Metabolism

What Is Metabolism?

Metabolism refers to the complex chemical reactions that occur within the cells of living organisms to maintain life. These metabolic processes are responsible for converting food into energy, building and repairing tissues, and managing waste products. Metabolism involves various biochemical reactions that are highly organized and regulated to sustain the body's functions.

There are two primary components of metabolism:

1. Anabolism is the set of metabolic pathways that build molecules and substances the body needs. It involves the synthesis of complex molecules from simpler ones, such as the formation of proteins from amino acids or the synthesis of new cellular components.

2. Catabolism is the set of metabolic pathways that break down larger molecules into smaller ones, releasing energy. Catabolic reactions are responsible for breaking